The Essential Foods Lists for Diabetes

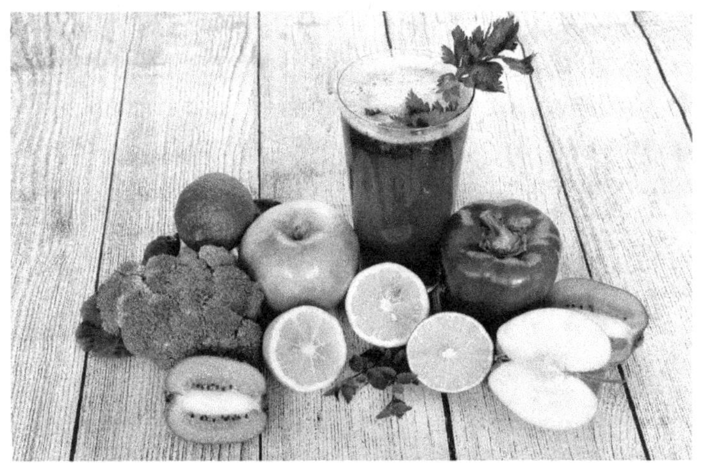

Your Comprehensive Guide to Managing Blood Sugar through Nutrition

Isaac Hendricks

Table of Contents

INTRODUCTION

Brief Overview of Diabetes and its impact on Nutrition

Diabetes is a chronic condition in which the body either does not create enough insulin or does not use it adequately. This results in high levels of glucose in the blood, which can lead to serious health complications if not managed properly.

Nutrition plays a crucial role in managing diabetes, as certain foods can affect blood sugar levels and overall health. People with diabetes are often advised to follow a balanced diet that includes plenty of fruits, vegetables, whole grains, lean proteins, and healthy fats. They must also monitor their carbohydrate intake, as carbohydrates have the biggest impact on blood sugar levels.

It is important for individuals with diabetes to work closely with a healthcare provider or registered dietitian to develop a Personalised nutrition plan that meets their specific needs and helps them manage their condition effectively. By making healthy food choices and monitoring their blood sugar levels regularly, individuals with diabetes can better control their condition and reduce their risk of complications.

Importance of Following a Diabetes-Friendly Diet

Following a diabetes-friendly diet is crucial for managing blood sugar levels and preventing complications associated with diabetes. Here are some key reasons why it is important to follow a diabetes-friendly diet:

1. Blood sugar control:

Eating a balanced diet that is low in sugar and carbohydrates helps regulate blood sugar levels. This is essential for individuals with diabetes to prevent spikes or drops in blood glucose levels, which can lead to serious health complications.

2. Weight management:

Maintaining a healthy weight is important for managing diabetes. A diabetes-friendly diet can help individuals control their calorie intake, leading to weight loss or maintenance. This, in turn, can improve insulin sensitivity and overall health.

3. Cardiovascular health:

Diabetes increases the risk of developing heart disease and other cardiovascular conditions. A diet rich in fruits, vegetables, whole grains, lean proteins, and healthy fats can help reduce the risk of heart disease by improving cholesterol levels and lowering blood pressure.

4. Energy levels:

Eating a balanced diet that includes complex carbohydrates and protein can help stabilise energy levels throughout the day. This is important for individuals with diabetes who may experience fluctuations in blood sugar levels that can lead to fatigue and other issues.

5. Nutrient absorption:

People with diabetes may have difficulty absorbing certain nutrients due to the condition. Following a diabetes-friendly diet that includes a variety of nutrient-dense foods can help ensure that the body is getting the necessary vitamins and minerals it needs to function properly.

In conclusion, following a diabetes-friendly diet is essential for managing blood sugar levels, promoting overall health, and reducing the risk of complications associated with diabetes. It is important for individuals with diabetes to work with a healthcare provider or a registered dietitian to create a customised meal plan that meets their nutritional needs and helps them maintain a healthy lifestyle.

Purpose and Structure of This Guide

- Purpose:

The purpose of this guide is to provide individuals with diabetes a comprehensive list of essential foods that they should include in their diet. The guide aims to educate and inform individuals about the nutritional value of different foods and how they can manage their blood sugar levels through dietary choices. The guide also provides tips on meal planning, portion control, and healthy eating habits that can help individuals with diabetes maintain a healthy lifestyle.

- Structure:

The guide is structured into different sections that cover various aspects of dietary management for individuals with diabetes. The sections are as follows: 1) Introduction, 2) Understanding Diabetes, 3) Essential Foods for Diabetes, 4) Meal Planning and Portion Control, and 5) Healthy Eating Habits. Each section is further divided into subsections that provide detailed information on the topic at hand. The guide also includes visual aids such as infographics, charts, and images to make the information more accessible and engaging.

Section 1: Introduction

This section provides an overview of the guide and its purpose. It explains the importance of dietary management for individuals with diabetes and how this guide can help them make informed choices about their food intake.

Section 2: Understanding Diabetes

This section provides a brief overview of diabetes, its causes, and how it affects the body. It explains

the difference between type 1 and type 2 diabetes
and how dietary choices can impact blood sugar
levels.

Section 3: Essential Foods for Diabetes

This section is the heart of the guide and provides a
comprehensive list of essential foods that
individuals with diabetes should include in their diet.
The list is divided into different categories such as
fruits, vegetables, whole grains, lean proteins, and
healthy fats. Each category includes a list of
specific foods that are rich in nutrients and low in
sugar and carbohydrates.

Section 4: Meal Planning and Portion Control

This section provides tips on meal planning and
portion control for individuals with diabetes. It
explains the importance of planning meals in
advance and how to calculate portion sizes based
on individual needs. It also provides suggestions for
healthy meal ideas and snacks that can help
individuals manage their blood sugar levels.

Section 5: Healthy Eating Habits

This section provides tips on healthy eating habits
that can help individuals with diabetes maintain a
healthy lifestyle. It explains the importance of eating
regularly, staying hydrated, and avoiding processed
and sugary foods. It also provides suggestions for
healthy substitutions and alternatives that can help
individuals make healthier choices.

The guide concludes by summarising the key takeaways from each section and emphasising the importance of dietary management for individuals with diabetes. It encourages individuals to consult with their healthcare provider for Personalised dietary advice and to make gradual changes to their diet over time. The guide also provides resources for further information and support, including websites, books, and support groups.

CHAPTER ONE

Carbohydrate-Rich Foods

List of Carbohydrate-Rich Foods That are Diabetes-Friendly

If you have diabetes, managing your blood sugar levels is crucial for your overall health. While carbohydrates are an essential part of a balanced diet, some types of carbohydrates can cause spikes in blood sugar levels. However, there are plenty of diabetes-friendly carbohydrate sources that are rich in nutrients and can help you manage your blood sugar levels. Here are a few examples:

- Fruits: Many fruits are rich in carbohydrates, but some are better choices for people with diabetes than others. Berries like strawberries, raspberries, and blueberries are low in sugar and high in fibre, making them a great option. Apples, pears, and oranges are also good choices as they contain fibre and have a lower glycemic index than other fruits like bananas and grapes.

- Vegetables: Vegetables are a great source of carbohydrates and fibre. Leafy greens like spinach and kale are low in

carbohydrates and high in fibre, making
them an excellent choice. Sweet potatoes,
carrots, and beets are also good options as
they contain complex carbohydrates that
are digested slowly and won't cause a spike
in blood sugar levels.

- Whole grains: Whole grains like brown rice,
  quinoa, and whole wheat bread are rich in
  carbohydrates but also contain fibre and
  other nutrients. These foods are digested
  slowly and won't cause a spike in blood
  sugar levels.

- Legumes: Legumes like lentils, chickpeas,
  and black beans are a great source of
  carbohydrates and protein. They are also
  rich in fibre and other nutrients that can help
  manage blood sugar levels.

- Nuts and seeds: Nuts and seeds are a good
  source of carbohydrates and healthy fats.
  Almonds, walnuts, and chia seeds are all
  good choices as they contain fibre and other
  nutrients that can help manage blood sugar
  levels.

Remember to always consult with your healthcare
provider or a registered dietitian for Personalised
recommendations based on your specific needs
and diabetes management plan.

Serving Sizes and Recommended Frequency

Carbohydrate-rich foods are an essential part of a balanced diet for individuals with diabetes. They provide the body with energy and essential nutrients, but it is important to consume them in moderation to help manage blood sugar levels.

When it comes to serving sizes and recommended frequency for carbohydrate-rich foods, it is important to consider the individual's overall diet, lifestyle, and blood sugar control. The following are general recommendations for serving sizes and frequency of carbohydrate-rich foods in the essential foods list for diabetes:

1. Whole grains: Whole grains such as whole wheat bread, brown rice, quinoa, and oats are good sources of complex carbohydrates that provide sustained energy and essential nutrients. It is recommended to include 1-2 servings of whole grains in each meal. A serving size is typically 1 slice of bread, 1/2 cup of cooked rice or pasta, or 1/2 cup of cooked oatmeal.

2. Fruits: Fruits are a natural source of carbohydrates, fibre, and essential vitamins and minerals. It is recommended to include 2-4 servings of fruits in the daily diet. A serving size is typically one medium-sized fruit, 1/2 cup of sliced fruit, or 1/4 cup of dried fruit.

3. Vegetables: Vegetables are low in carbohydrates and provide essential nutrients, fibre, and antioxidants. It is recommended to include 3-5 servings of vegetables in the daily diet. A serving size is typically 1 cup of raw leafy greens or 1/2 cup of cooked vegetables.

4. Legumes: Legumes such as beans, lentils, and chickpeas are a good source of carbohydrates, protein, and fibre. It is recommended to include 1-2 servings of legumes in the daily diet. A serving size is typically 1/2 cup of cooked beans or lentils.

5. Dairy: Dairy products such as milk, yoghurt, and cheese provide carbohydrates, protein, calcium, and other essential nutrients. It is recommended to include 2-3 servings of dairy in the daily diet. A serving size is typically 1 cup of milk, 6-8 ounces of yoghurt, or 1-2 ounces of cheese.

It is important to work with a registered dietitian or healthcare provider to create a Personalised meal plan that takes into account individual nutritional needs, blood sugar levels, and medication management. Monitoring portion sizes, choosing whole foods, and balancing carbohydrate intake with other nutrients can help individuals with diabetes manage their condition effectively.

Tips for Managing Carbohydrate Intake

Managing carbohydrate intake is crucial for individuals with diabetes, as it helps to regulate blood sugar levels. Carbohydrate-rich foods, such as fruits, vegetables, grains, and dairy products, can be a part of a healthy diabetes diet when consumed in moderation and as part of a balanced meal plan. Here are some tips for managing carbohydrate intake for carbohydrate-rich foods:

1. Understand the glycemic index:

The glycemic index (GI) is a measure of how quickly a food raises blood sugar levels. Foods with a high GI, such as white bread and pasta, should be consumed in moderation, while foods with a low GI, such as whole-grain bread and oatmeal, are better choices.

2. Count carbohydrates:

Keeping track of the amount of carbohydrates you consume can help you manage your blood sugar levels. Use a food diary or an app to track your carb intake and adjust your meal plan accordingly. Aim for 45-60 grams of carbohydrates per meal. 3. Choose fibre-rich carbohydrates: Foods that are high in fibre, such as fruits, vegetables, and whole grains, are digested more slowly, which helps to prevent spikes in blood sugar levels.

Adding protein and healthy fats to your meals can help to slow down the absorption of carbohydrates, which can help to prevent blood sugar spikes. For example, pair a piece of fruit with a handful of nuts or a hard-boiled egg.

Processed and sugary foods, such as candy, soda, and baked goods, should be consumed in moderation, as they are high in carbohydrates and can cause rapid spikes in blood sugar levels.

A healthcare provider or a registered dietitian can help you develop a Personalised meal plan that meets your specific needs and goals. They can also provide guidance on how to manage carbohydrate intake and make healthy food choices.

By following these tips, individuals with diabetes can manage their carbohydrate intake and enjoy a variety of carbohydrate-rich foods as part of a healthy and balanced diet.

CHAPTER TWO

Protein-Rich Foods

List of Protein-Rich Foods That are Diabetes-Friendly

For individuals with diabetes, managing blood sugar levels through a balanced diet that includes protein-rich foods can be beneficial for overall health and weight management. Here is a list of protein-rich foods that are diabetes-friendly:

1. Eggs: A large egg contains approximately 6 grams of protein, making it an excellent source for people with diabetes. Eggs are also rich in vitamins and minerals, such as vitamin D, choline, and selenium.

2. Greek yoghourt: Greek yoghourt is high in protein, with a 6-ounce serving containing around 17 grams. It is also low in carbohydrates and sugar, making it a great option for people with diabetes.

3. Nuts and seeds: Almonds, pistachios, pumpkin seeds, and chia seeds are all high in protein and healthy fats. They also include fibre, which can help control blood sugar levels.

4. Lean meats: Chicken, turkey, and fish are all low in fat and calories, making them excellent sources of protein for people with diabetes. A 3-ounce serving of chicken breast contains approximately 27 grams of protein.

5. Lentils: Lentils are a great source of plant-based protein, with a 1/2 cup serving containing around 9 grams. They are also high in fibre and other nutrients, such as iron and folate.

6. Tofu: Tofu is a versatile source of protein, with a 3-ounce serving containing around 8 grams. It is also low in calories and fat, making it a great option for people with diabetes.

7. Quinoa: Quinoa is a gluten-free grain that is high in protein, with a 1/2 cup serving containing around 4 grams. It is also rich in fibre, vitamins, and minerals.

8. Cottage cheese: Cottage cheese is a good source of protein, with a 1/2 cup serving containing around 14 grams. It is also low in carbohydrates and sugar, making it a great option for people with diabetes.

9. Edamame: Edamame is a soybean that is high in protein, with a 1/2 cup serving containing around 8 grams. It is also rich in fibre, vitamins, and minerals.

10. Peanut butter: Peanut butter is a good source of protein, with a 2-tablespoon serving containing around 7 grams. It is also rich in healthy fats and fibre, making it a great option for people with diabetes.

Incorporating these protein-rich foods into a diabetes-friendly diet can help manage blood sugar levels, promote weight loss, and improve overall health. It's essential to remember to monitor portion sizes and consult with a healthcare professional or registered dietitian for Personalised dietary recommendations.

Serving Sizes and Recommended Frequency

Protein-rich foods play an essential role in managing diabetes as they help regulate blood sugar levels and promote feelings of fullness. However, it's crucial to consume these foods in appropriate serving sizes and frequencies to reap their benefits without overdoing it. Here's a guide to serving sizes and recommended frequencies for protein-rich foods for people with diabetes:

Serving sizes:

- Beans and legumes: A serving size is about 1/2 cup (cooked) or 1/4 cup of dried beans or legumes. This amount provides around seven grams of protein for people with diabetes who follow a vegetarian diet or around five grams for those who follow a non-vegetarian diet.

- Nuts and seeds: A serving size is about 1/4 cup or 30 grams. This amount provides around seven grams of protein for people with diabetes who follow a vegetarian diet or around five grams for those who follow a non-vegetarian diet.

- Eggs: A serving size is about one large egg for people with diabetes who follow a non-vegetarian diet. This amount provides around six grams of protein for people with diabetes who follow a non-vegetarian diet or around four grams for those who follow a vegetarian diet (as vegetarians may opt for plant-based protein sources instead).

- Dairy products: A serving size is about one cup (245 grams) for people with diabetes who follow a non-vegetarian diet or about one cup (250 millilitres) for people with diabetes who follow a vegetarian diet. This amount provides around eight grams of protein for people with diabetes who follow a non-vegetarian diet or around six grams for those who follow a vegetarian diet (as vegetarians may opt for plant-based protein sources instead).

- Meat and poultry: A serving size is about three to four oz (85-113 grams) for people with diabetes who follow a non-vegetarian diet (equivalent to about one deck of cards). This amount provides around seven grams of protein for people with diabetes who follow a non-vegetarian diet or around five grams for those who follow a vegetarian diet (as vegetarians may opt for plant-based protein sources instead).

Recommended Frequencies:

- ☐ Beans and legumes: People with diabetes should aim to consume about 1/2 to 1 cup (cooked) of beans or legumes per day.

- ☐ Nuts and seeds: People with diabetes should aim to consume about 1/4 to 1/2 cup (30-60 grams) of nuts or seeds daily as part of a balanced diet that includes other food groups in appropriate proportions.

- ☐ Eggs: People with diabetes can consume eggs as part of a balanced diet that includes other food groups in appropriate proportions (either one large egg daily for non-vegetarians or plant-based protein sources for vegetarians).

- ☐ Dairy products: People with diabetes should aim to consume about one to two cups

(245-250 millilitres) of low-fat dairy products daily as part of a balanced diet that includes other food groups in appropriate proportions (either one cup daily for non-vegetarians or plant-based alternatives for vegetarians).

- ☐ Meat and poultry: People with diabetes should aim to consume about three to four oz (85-113 grams) of lean meat or poultry daily as part of a balanced diet that includes other food groups in appropriate proportions (either three to four oz daily for non-vegetarians or plant-based protein sources for vegetarians).

In summary, people with diabetes should aim to consume a variety of protein-rich foods in appropriate serving sizes and frequencies to manage blood sugar levels and promote overall health.
Consulting a healthcare provider or a registered dietitian can provide personalised recommendations based on individual needs and preferences.

Tips for Managing Protein Intake

Managing protein intake is crucial for individuals with diabetes as it helps regulate blood sugar levels, builds and repairs tissues, and promotes overall health. Protein-rich foods are an essential part of a balanced diet for people with diabetes, but it's crucial to consume them in moderation to prevent excess calories and potential complications. Here are some tips for managing protein intake for protein-rich foods in the essential foods lists for diabetes:

Choose lean sources of protein:

Opt for lean sources of protein such as chicken breast, turkey breast, fish, beans, lentils, and low-fat dairy products. These foods are lower in calories and fat than red meat or processed meats like sausage or bacon. They also provide necessary amino acids for muscle growth and repair.

Portion control:

It's essential to watch portion sizes when consuming protein-rich foods as they can be high in calories. A serving size of protein is typically 3-4 ounces, which is about the size of a deck of cards.

Spread protein intake throughout the day:

Consuming protein evenly throughout the day can help prevent spikes in blood sugar levels. Aim to include protein at every meal and snack to keep blood sugar levels stable. This can also help prevent overeating and promote satiety.

Pair protein with fibre:

Pairing protein with fibre-rich foods like whole grains, vegetables, and fruits can help slow down the digestion process, preventing blood sugar spikes. This also helps keep you fuller for longer, preventing overeating.

Limit processed and high-fat protein sources:

Processed and high-fat protein sources like sausage, bacon, and fatty cuts of meat should be consumed in moderation. These foods are often high in calories, saturated fat, and sodium, which can contribute to weight gain, high cholesterol, and high blood pressure.

Consult a healthcare provider or a registered dietitian:

It's essential to consult a healthcare provider or a registered dietitian to develop a personalised meal plan that meets your specific dietary needs and goals. They can provide guidance on portion sizes, food choices, and meal planning to help manage blood sugar levels and promote overall health.

CHAPTER THREE

Fat-Rich Foods

List of Fat-Rich Foods That are Diabetes-Friendly

If you have diabetes, managing your blood sugar levels is crucial to maintaining good health. While it's important to limit your intake of foods high in sugar and carbohydrates, you may still enjoy foods that are rich in healthy fats. Here's a list of fat-rich foods that are diabetes-friendly:

1. Avocado: This fruit is high in monounsaturated fats, which can help improve cholesterol levels and reduce the risk of heart disease. Avocado is also rich in fibre and nutrients like potassium and vitamin C.

2. Nuts and seeds: Almonds, walnuts, chia seeds, and flaxseeds are all excellent sources of healthy fats, protein, and fibre. They can be enjoyed as a snack or added to salads, oatmeal, or yoghurt.

3. Fatty fish: Salmon, mackerel, and sardines are all rich in omega-3 fatty acids, which can help reduce inflammation and lower the

risk of heart disease. These fish are also a good source of protein and other nutrients.

4. Olive oil: This healthy fat is a staple in the Mediterranean diet and is rich in monounsaturated fats. It can be used as a dressing for salads, drizzled over vegetables, or used to sauté foods.

5. Coconut oil: While coconut oil is high in saturated fat, it's also rich in medium-chain triglycerides (MCTs), which can help boost energy levels and promote weight loss. It's best to use coconut oil in moderation and in place of other sources of saturated fat.

6. Dark chocolate: While it's important to enjoy chocolate in moderation, dark chocolate is a good source of healthy fats and antioxidants. Look for chocolate with at least 70% cocoa to reap the health benefits.

Remember to always consult with a healthcare provider or a registered dietitian for personalised nutrition advice based on your individual needs and health condition.

Serving Sizes and Recommended Frequency

When it comes to managing diabetes, it's crucial to pay close attention to the types and amounts of food consumed. While carbohydrates and sugar intake are often the primary focus, fat-rich foods also play a significant role in maintaining blood sugar levels. Here, we'll discuss serving sizes and recommended frequency for fat-rich foods in The Essential Foods Lists for Diabetes.

First and foremost, it is critical to recognize that not all fats are created equal. Some fats, like saturated and trans fats, can increase the risk of heart disease and negatively impact blood sugar control. On the other hand, unsaturated fats, such as monounsaturated and polyunsaturated fats, can help lower cholesterol levels and improve blood sugar management.

The American Diabetes Association recommends that people with diabetes aim for 20-35% of their daily calories to come from fat. This equates to approximately 44-77 grams of fat per day for a 2,000-calorie diet.

Here are some recommended serving sizes for fat-rich foods:

1. Nuts and Seeds: A serving size is approximately 1/4 cup (32 grams) or 1 ounce (28 grams). Nuts and seeds are rich in healthy fats, fibre, and protein, making them a great snack option for people with diabetes.

2. Avocado: A serving size is approximately 1/3 avocado (57 grams). Avocado is high in monounsaturated fats, fibre, and potassium, making it a nutritious addition to any meal.

3. Olive Oil: A serving size is approximately 1 tablespoon (14 grams). Olive oil is rich in monounsaturated fats and can be used as a healthy substitute for butter or margarine in cooking and baking.

4. Fatty Fish: A serving size is approximately 3 ounces (85 grams) cooked. Fatty fish, such as salmon, mackerel, and sardines, are rich in omega-3 fatty acids, which can help improve heart health and blood sugar control.

5. Cheese: A serving size is approximately 1 ounce (28 grams) or 1 slice. Cheese is high in fat and calories, so it should be consumed in moderation as part of a balanced meal.

When it comes to recommended frequency, it's essential to incorporate fat-rich foods into a balanced meal plan. Here are some guidelines:

1. Nuts and Seeds: Enjoy a serving of nuts or seeds as a snack or add them to a salad or oatmeal for added crunch and healthy fats.

2. Avocado: Add avocado to sandwiches, salads, or as a dip for vegetables.

3. Olive Oil: Use olive oil as a healthy substitute for butter or margarine in cooking and baking.

4. Fatty Fish: Incorporate fatty fish into your diet 2-3 times per week.

5. Cheese: Enjoy a serving of cheese as part of a balanced meal, such as a cheese and vegetable omelette or a cheese and whole-grain cracker snack.

In conclusion, while fat-rich foods should be consumed in moderation, they can be a part of a healthy and balanced diet for people with diabetes. By following the recommended serving sizes and incorporating these foods into a balanced meal plan, individuals with diabetes can enjoy the health benefits of healthy fats while managing their blood sugar levels.

Tips for Managing Fat Intake

Managing fat intake is crucial for individuals with diabetes, as it can impact their blood sugar levels and overall health. Here are some tips for managing fat intake when consuming fat-rich foods from the essential foods list for diabetes:

- Choose healthy fats: Opt for sources of unsaturated fats such as avocados, nuts, seeds, and olive oil instead of saturated fats found in red meat, butter, and full-fat dairy products. Healthy fats can help improve cholesterol levels and reduce the risk of heart disease.

- Pay attention to portion sizes: Even healthy fats contain calories, so it's important to monitor your portion sizes. Be mindful of serving sizes when consuming nuts, seeds, nut butter, and oils to avoid overeating.

- Limit processed and fried foods: Avoid foods that are high in trans fats, such as fried foods, pastries, and packaged snacks. These fats can increase inflammation and insulin resistance, putting individuals with diabetes at greater risk for complications.

- Read food labels: Check the nutrition labels on packaged foods to identify the amount of saturated and trans fats they contain. Choose products with lower saturated fat content, and aim to limit trans fats as much as possible.

- Balance your meals: Include a variety of nutrient-dense foods in your meals to ensure you're getting a balance of carbohydrates, proteins, and fats. Incorporate lean proteins, whole grains, fruits, vegetables, and healthy fats to create well-rounded meals that support blood sugar management.

- Cook at home: By preparing meals at home, you have more control over the ingredients and cooking methods used. Use healthier cooking techniques such as grilling, baking, steaming, or sautéing with minimal oil to limit your fat intake.

- Snack mindfully: When choosing snacks, opt for whole foods like fresh fruits, vegetables, Greek yoghurt, or a handful of nuts instead of processed snacks like chips or cookies. These options provide essential nutrients without the excess saturated and trans fats.

- Be mindful of hidden fats: Some foods may contain hidden fats, such as dairy products, salad dressings, sauces, and baked goods. Make sure to read ingredient lists and choose low-fat or fat-free alternatives when possible.

By incorporating these tips into your meal planning and food choices, you can effectively manage your fat intake while enjoying a diverse and Flavourful diet that supports your diabetes management goals. It's essential to work with a healthcare provider or dietitian to create a personalised nutrition plan tailored to your individual needs and preferences.

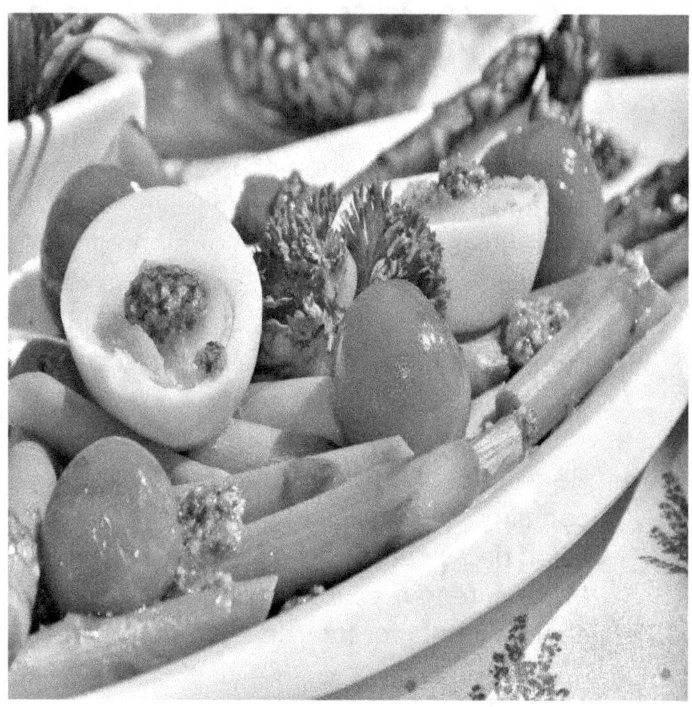

CHAPTER FOUR

Foods to Limit or Avoid

List of Foods That Should Be Limited or Avoided in a Diabetes-Friendly Diet

Sugary drinks:

These include soda, fruit juice, sports drinks, and flavoured water. They are high in added sugars and can cause a rapid spike in blood sugar levels.

Processed foods:

These are often high in added sugars, salt, and unhealthy fats. Examples include candy, cookies, cakes, and packaged snacks like chips and crackers.

White bread and pasta:

These are made with refined flour and have a high glycemic index (GI), which can cause a rapid rise in blood sugar levels. Opt for whole-grain bread and pasta instead to help manage blood sugar levels more effectively.

Fried foods:

These are often high in unhealthy fats and calories and can lead to weight gain, which can worsen diabetes management.

High-fat dairy products:

These include whole milk, cream, and cheese with a high fat content. Instead, choose low-fat or fat-free dairy products.

Processed meats:

These include bacon, sausage, and deli meats, which are often high in sodium and unhealthy fats. Choose lean cuts of meat and prepare them in healthy ways, such as grilling or baking.

Alcohol:

While moderate alcohol consumption may be acceptable for some people with diabetes, it's essential to be aware of the calories and sugar content in alcoholic beverages.

High-sugar fruits:

While fruits are generally healthy, some fruits like pineapple, mango, and bananas are high in sugar. It's best to consume them in moderation and pair them with other low-GI foods to help manage blood sugar levels.

Coconut and palm oil:

These oils are high in saturated fats and should be consumed in moderation.

Salt:

While salt is essential for maintaining fluid balance, too much salt can lead to high blood pressure, which is a risk factor for diabetes complications. Limit salt intake and opt for herbs and spices to add flavour to your meals.

It's essential to work with a healthcare provider or a registered dietitian to develop a Personalised diabetes management plan that takes into account individual needs and preferences. By making informed food choices and managing blood sugar levels effectively, people with diabetes can enjoy a healthy and fulfilling lifestyle.

Reasons for Avoiding or Limiting These Foods

As someone with diabetes, it's essential to manage your blood sugar levels to prevent complications. While a healthy diet is crucial for diabetes management, some foods should be limited or avoided altogether. Here are some reasons why:

- Sugary drinks and foods: Consuming too much sugar can cause a rapid spike in blood sugar levels, followed by a crash. This can lead to hunger, fatigue, and mood swings. Limiting sugary drinks and foods, such as soda, candy, and baked goods, can help regulate blood sugar levels.

- Processed foods: Processed foods, such as packaged snacks, fast food, and frozen meals, are often high in sodium, unhealthy fats, and added sugars. These foods can lead to weight gain, high blood pressure, and high cholesterol levels, which can increase the risk of diabetes complications.

- Saturated and trans fats: Saturated and trans fats can increase LDL (bad) cholesterol levels, which can lead to heart disease. Foods high in these fats include fried foods, processed meats, and baked goods made with hydrogenated oils. Limiting these foods can help reduce the risk of heart disease.

- Alcohol: While alcohol can lower blood sugar levels, it can also cause a sudden drop in blood sugar levels, known as hypoglycemia. This can be dangerous, especially if you're taking diabetes medication. Limiting alcohol intake or avoiding it altogether can help prevent hypoglycemia.

- High-fat meats: High-fat meats, such as bacon, sausage, and fatty cuts of beef, can be high in saturated fats and cholesterol. These foods can increase the risk of heart disease and should be limited.

- Salt: A high-salt diet can lead to high blood pressure, which can increase the risk of diabetes complications. Limiting salt intake and choosing low-sodium options can help regulate blood pressure.

Remember, a healthy diet is essential for diabetes management, but it's also important to enjoy a variety of foods in moderation. Consult with a healthcare provider or a registered dietitian for Personalised dietary recommendations.

Tips for Making Healthier Choice

As someone with diabetes, making healthy food choices is crucial in managing blood sugar levels. While some foods are essential for a balanced diet, others should be limited or avoided altogether due to their high sugar, carbohydrate, or fat content. Here are some tips for making healthier choices when it comes to foods to limit or avoid in your diabetes meal plan:

1. Limit processed and packaged foods:
Processed and packaged foods often contain added sugars, salt, and unhealthy fats. Instead, opt for whole, unprocessed foods such as fresh fruits, vegetables, whole grains, and lean proteins.

2. Watch out for hidden sugars: Many foods that you might not expect, such as sauces, dressings, and condiments, can be high in sugar. Read labels carefully and choose products with lower sugar content.

3. Limit sugary drinks: Sugary drinks like soda, juice, and sports drinks can cause a rapid spike in blood sugar levels. Instead, choose water, unsweetened tea, or sparkling water with a slice of lemon or lime for flavour.

4. Choose low-fat dairy products: Dairy products like cheese, yoghurt, and milk can be a good source of protein and calcium, but choose low-fat or fat-free options to limit saturated fat intake.

5. Watch portion sizes: Even healthy foods can be high in calories and carbohydrates if consumed in large portions. Practice portion control by using smaller plates or measuring out servings with a food scale or measuring cups.

6. Limit alcohol intake: Alcohol can cause a rapid drop in blood sugar levels followed by a rebound spike. If you choose to drink, do so in moderation and pair it with a meal to help slow down the absorption of alcohol.

7. Choose healthy fats: While it's important to limit saturated fats, healthy fats like those found in avocados, nuts, seeds, olive oil, and fatty fish like salmon can help keep you feeling fuller longer while providing essential nutrients.

8. Be mindful of carbohydrate intake: Carbohydrates can cause a rapid rise in blood sugar levels, so it's important to be mindful of how

many carbs you're consuming in a meal or snack.
Choose complex carbohydrates like whole grains,
fruits, and vegetables over simple carbohydrates
like candy, white bread, and pastries.

Remember, making healthy food choices is an
ongoing process, and it's okay to indulge in
moderation. The key is to find a balance that works
for you and your diabetes management plan.
Consult with a registered dietitian or healthcare
provider for Personalised guidance on creating a
healthy meal plan.

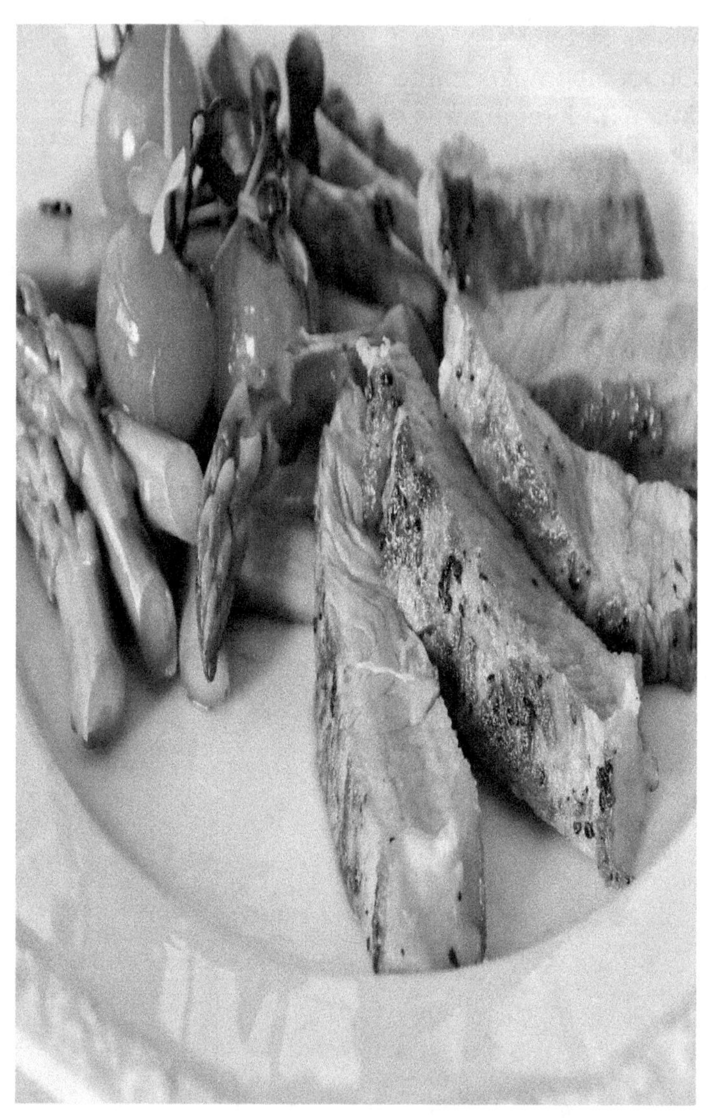

CHAPTER FIVE

Meal Planning and Preparation Tips

Strategies for Planning Diabetes-Friendly Meals

Planning diabetes-friendly meals can help you manage your blood sugar levels and ensure you are eating a balanced and nutritious diet. Here are some strategies to help you plan and prepare diabetes-friendly meals:

1. Focus on the essential foods for diabetes: When planning your meals, refer to the essential foods lists for diabetes, which include foods such as lean proteins, whole grains, fruits, vegetables, and healthy fats. These foods can help you keep your blood sugar levels stable and provide you with important nutrients.

2. Portion control: It's important to pay attention to portion sizes when planning your meals. Use measuring cups or a food scale to ensure that you are consuming the proper amount of each food group. Portion control can help you manage your blood sugar levels and maintain a healthy weight.

3. Incorporate a variety of foods: To ensure
    you are getting a well-balanced diet, include
    a variety of foods in your meals. Aim to
    include a source of protein, whole grains,
    fruits, vegetables, and healthy fats in each
    meal. This will help you get a mix of
    important nutrients and keep your blood
    sugar levels stable.

4. Plan ahead: Take the time to plan your
    meals for the week to ensure you have all
    the ingredients you need on hand. Planning
    ahead can help you avoid last-minute
    decisions that may not be as healthy.
    Consider using a meal planning app or
    writing out a weekly meal plan to stay
    organised.

5. Prepare meals in advance: To save time
    during the week, consider preparing some
    meals in advance. You can cook large
    batches of food and portion them out for
    easy meals throughout the week. This can
    help you avoid unhealthy takeout options
    when you are short on time.

6. Make simple swaps: When preparing meals,
    look for opportunities to make simple swaps
    to lower the calories or carbohydrates in a
    dish. For example, you can use whole
    wheat pasta instead of regular pasta, or opt

for grilled chicken instead of fried chicken. Small changes can add up to big benefits for your health.

By following these strategies for planning and preparing diabetes-friendly meals, you can ensure you are eating a balanced and nutritious diet that will help you manage your blood sugar levels and improve your overall health. Remember to consult with a healthcare provider or registered dietitian for personalised guidance on managing your diabetes through diet.

Tips for Preparing Meals That are Both Healthy and Delicious

Preparing meals can be challenging when trying to balance health concerns with taste preferences. For individuals with diabetes, it's essential to focus on meals that are both healthy and delicious. Here are some meal planning and preparation techniques that may be helpful:

Start with a balanced plate:

Aim for a plate that is half filled with non-starchy vegetables, one-quarter with a lean protein source, and one-quarter with a whole grain or starchy vegetable. By following this guideline, you can ensure you're getting a variety of nutrients while keeping portion sizes in check.

Use healthy cooking methods:

Grilling, baking, steaming or roasting your food instead of frying can help reduce the amount of unhealthy fats and calories in your meals. Try experimenting with different seasonings and marinades to add flavour without adding excess salt or sugar.

Incorporate healthy fats:

While it's essential to limit saturated and trans fats, healthy fats like avocados, nuts, seeds, olive oil or fatty fish can help you feel fuller for longer periods. Try adding a handful of nuts to your salad or using olive oil to dress your veggies.

Watch your portion sizes:

It's easy to overeat, especially when you're enjoying delicious food. Use smaller plates, measure out your servings, and pay attention to your hunger and fullness cues.

Get creative with spices:

Spices like cumin or turmeric can add flavour to your meals while also providing health benefits. Experiment with several spice mixtures to see what you like best. Just remember to use them in moderation as some spices can be high in sodium.

Don't forget about desserts:

You don't have to give up your sweet tooth entirely. Try incorporating healthier dessert options like fresh fruit or dark chocolate into your meal plan. Just make sure to enjoy them in moderation.

Meal planning can help you stay on track with your healthy eating goals. Spend some time each week planning out your meals and snacks, as well as creating a grocery list. This can help you avoid impulse buys and ensure you have all the ingredients you need on hand.

By following these tips, you can create meals that are both healthy and delicious. Remember to always consult with your healthcare provider or a registered dietitian for Personalised meal planning advice.

Suggestions for Incorporating Variety and Flavour into Your Diet

Incorporating variety and flavour into your diet is essential for maintaining a healthy and balanced meal plan, especially if you have diabetes. Here are some suggestions for meal planning and preparation tips:

1. **Include a variety of foods:** Eating a wide range of foods can help ensure that you're getting all the nutrients your body needs. Aim to include fruits, vegetables, whole grains, lean proteins, and healthy fats in each meal.

2. **Experiment with spices and herbs:** Adding flavorful spices and herbs can make your meals more interesting and delicious without adding extra calories or sugar. Try using cinnamon, cumin, garlic, or ginger in your cooking.

3. **Use healthy fats:** Incorporate healthy fats like avocado, nuts, and olive oil into your meals to add flavour and richness. These fats can also help you feel fuller and satisfied.

4. **Try new foods:** Don't be afraid to try new fruits, vegetables, and whole grains that you've never had before. This can help you discover new flavours and textures that you enjoy.

5. **Make healthy swaps:** Instead of using sugar or processed sauces, try using natural sweeteners like honey or maple syrup,

CONCLUSION

Summary of Key Points Covered in This Guide

In this guide for managing diabetes through diet, several key points have been covered.

Firstly, it is essential to maintain a healthy weight and engage in regular physical activity to manage blood sugar levels.

Secondly, a balanced diet rich in fibre, protein, and healthy fats is recommended to prevent spikes in blood sugar.

Thirdly, it is crucial to limit the intake of foods with a high glycemic index, such as sugary drinks, white bread, and processed snacks, as they can cause rapid increases in blood sugar.

Fourthly, incorporating foods with a low glycemic index, such as whole grains, fruits, and vegetables, can help regulate blood sugar levels.

Lastly, it is essential to monitor blood sugar levels regularly and consult with a healthcare provider or a registered dietitian for Personalised dietary recommendations based on individual needs and preferences.

By following these key points, individuals with diabetes can manage their condition effectively and improve their overall health and well-being.

Encouragement to Consult with a Healthcare Provider or Registered Dietitian for Personalised Nutrition Advice

As we come to the end of our discussion on essential foods for managing diabetes, it's crucial to emphasise the importance of consulting with a healthcare provider or registered dietitian for Personalised nutrition advice. While this list provides a general guideline, individual needs and circumstances may require tailored recommendations.

A healthcare provider or registered dietitian can help individuals with diabetes create a meal plan that takes into account factors such as medication, blood sugar levels, lifestyle, and personal preferences. They can provide guidance on portion sizes, meal timing, and strategies for managing blood sugar during and after meals.

Moreover, a healthcare provider or registered dietitian can help individuals with diabetes identify potential nutritional deficiencies, such as vitamin D, calcium, or magnesium, and recommend supplements or dietary modifications to address them. They can also provide education on healthy cooking techniques, label reading, and restaurant dining tips to help individuals make informed choices while eating out.

In conclusion, while this list provides valuable insights into essential foods for managing diabetes, it's essential to remember that individual needs and circumstances may require Personalised nutrition advice. Consulting with a healthcare provider or registered dietitian can provide tailored recommendations, guidance, and support to help individuals with diabetes manage their condition effectively.

Resources for Further Information and Support

If you are living with diabetes, it's essential to make informed choices about your diet to manage your blood sugar levels. The Essential Foods Lists for Diabetes is a helpful resource that provides a guide to healthy food options for people with diabetes. However, there is always more to learn about diabetes management, and here we've compiled a list of additional resources for further information and support:

1. American Diabetes Association (ADA):

The ADA is a leading organisation dedicated to diabetes research, education and advocacy. Their website offers a wealth of information on diabetes management, including healthy eating tips, recipes, and resources for finding a diabetes educator.

2. Diabetes.org:

This website, run by the American Diabetes Association, provides a wide range of resources for people with diabetes, including articles on nutrition, exercise, and diabetes technology.

3. National Institute of Diabetes and Digestive and Kidney Diseases (NIDDK):

This government organisation provides information on diabetes research, treatment, and management, as well as resources for finding diabetes care providers.

4. MyPlate:

This website, run by the USDA, provides a simple guide to healthy eating based on four food groups: fruits, vegetables, grains, and protein. It includes tips on portion sizes, healthy meal planning, recipes, cooking videos, grocery lists and more. It's a great resource to help people with diabetes make healthy food choices.

5. Diabeat:

This app, developed by a team of healthcare professionals, provides Personalised meal plans, recipes, and nutrition advice based on individual diabetes management goals. It also includes features like a food diary, blood sugar tracking, medication reminders, and more. It's a convenient and helpful tool for people with diabetes who want to manage their diet and blood sugar levels more effectively.

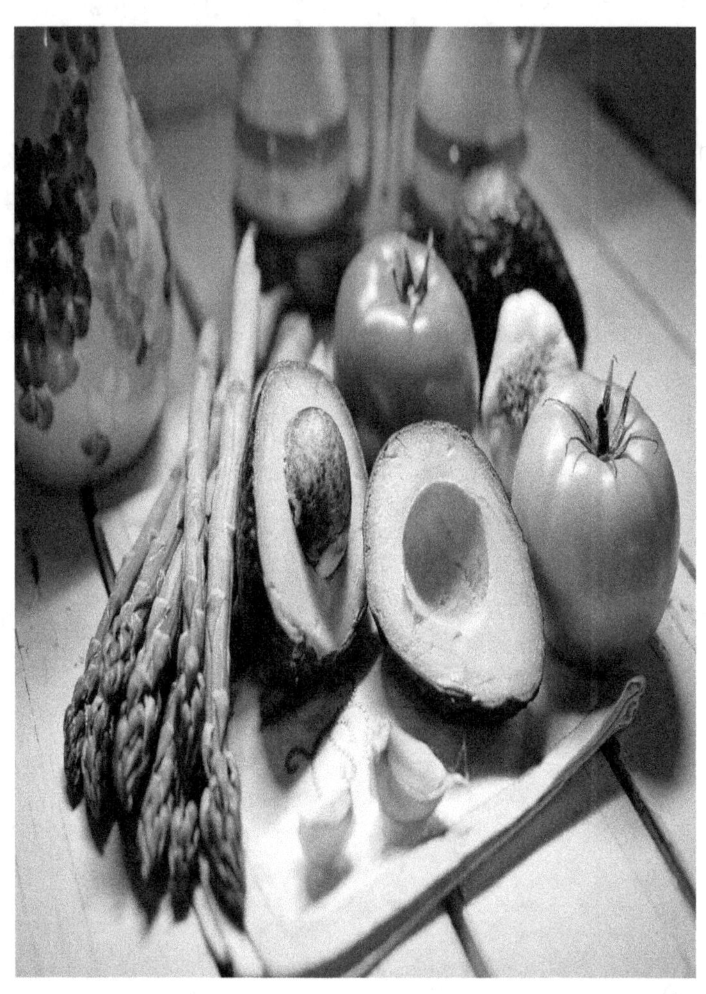